# 7 Secrets to Living

# Raw Foods

Shifting your Food Paradigms
for Easy, Simple, Healthy Eating

Allie Kent
Raw Food Chef & Instructor

To David,

In taking care of yourself,
may this brief tome
assist you to achieve
your most vibrant
health!

— Chef Allie

Moxie Publishing
5644 Westheimer Rd., #473
Houston, TX  77056

For more information, contact:
info@rawmmgood.com

Cover Design:  Manjari Handerson,
www.manjarigraphics.com
Editing: Andrea M. Sattinger,
The Sattinger Group


Library of Congress Control Number:
2009907626

Kent, Allie.
   7 Secrets to Living Raw Foods /
   Allie Kent. – 1st ed.

ISBN-13: 978-0-9824309-0-3
ISBN-10: 0-9824309-0-6

   1.   Health. 2. Food 3. Raw Food

   First Edition: August 2009

## Dedication

I dedicate this book to the Universal Spirit
of us all, and in us all, in unbounded
Gratitude.

Special Mention for two dear friends:
- Stacey Mayo,
  www.balancedliving.com, for her
  encouragement and suggestions
- Cornelia Powell,
  www.corneliapowell.com, for proof
  reading and her suggestions

## Acknowledgments

I wish to express my heartfelt gratitude to all who have gone before me on the Raw Foods pathway. And, because they were particularly helpful in my learning, I would like to make special mention of appreciation to:

* Dr. Fred Bisci, via his CD, *Raw Food and Science: 30 Years of Raw*
* Victoria Boutenko, via her book *Green for Life*
* Alissa Cohen, via her book *Living on Live Foods*, and her certification training
* Gabriel Cousens M.D., via his books *Rainbow Green Live-Food Cuisine* and *Conscious Eating*
* Amanda Crook, who started my raw chef trainings off right with her excitement and service to all in the classes she taught
* Chef Ito at Au Lac in Orange County, California, and Chef Matthew Kenney of New York City, via several venues; both Chefs inspire me with their creativity, and the way they consistently offer in their restaurants overall, high-grade, delectable raw foods
* Paul Nison, via his book *The Raw Life*
* Diane Olive, who was one of the first to introduce me to raw foods and model this lifestyle for me when I lived in San Diego, as well as via her book *Think Before You Eat*
* Cherie Soria, under whom I trained at her school *Living Light Culinary Arts Institute* in Fort Bragg, California

## About the Author

Many people struggle with their weight, and find themselves living with a general lack of energy or health problems. But many of these conditions and diseases, including diabetes, high blood pressure, and extreme fatigue can be reversed by making a few relatively easy changes.

I help people learn a different way to eat well: to eat foods that satisfy and taste good, and to learn how to prepare foods in ways that best help us attain a healthy weight, and gain the energy and health we all seek.

I teach people about fresh, whole, plant-based, foods, and how to prepare them.

I have personally experienced the exhaustion of being more than 65 pounds overweight; I have known the yo-yo cycle of dieting and taking the diet supplements that are widely advertised on the market, and I have seen the impacts of this on my health. In 2004, I changed my life; I fully adopted a lifestyle of eating living foods. Later, however, I experienced the discernment that comes with making a change, then failing, and then finally adopting the change as a way of life. I was so excited by what I discovered, that I sought Raw Chef training, and became a certified Living Foods Instructor.

If you're interested in hearing more of the inspiration and motivation that got me to where I am today (a svelte 127 pounds), then read on and find out how you can start your own healthy life journey…

You can find out more about Allie and her Raw Food resources at: www.rawmmgood.com

## SPECIAL OFFER:

If you will go to my website, www.rawmmgood.com , and "contact me" with your contact information, I will send you a special one week [5 days] Living Foods menu plan, including recipes and shopping list. Be sure to type in "SPECIAL MENU" in the subject line.

To share this book with others and/or purchase it in bulk, go to my web-store at:

www.rawmmgood.com

Also available via my store, are high-grade essential oils, herbs, food, and specialty kitchen items.

And, I invite you to join me on-line via:

- Facebook – http://www.facebook.com/chefallie
- Twitter – http://twitter.com/allieraw

# Secret #1:

## Intention

- Commitment, and
- Staying Curious

**"If we truly want to create a life that is grounded in basic well-being, we must decide to commit ourselves to learning what it takes to thrive instead of merely survive."** ~ Susan Velasquez

**"Commitment unlocks the doors of imagination, allows vision, and gives us the "right stuff" to turn our dreams into reality."** ~ James Womack

The first secret to easily living a simple, healthy raw food lifestyle is to state your intent; better yet, put it in writing, placing it somewhere that you can view it every day. With your commitment to continue applying the concepts you learn here, even when you may slip away from your intended goal, you will ultimately succeed.

Data from the Centers for Disease Control and Prevention show that 66% of American adults are overweight and of those, 32% are obese. These numbers have been on the rise for over 25 years.

The American Dietetic Association (ADA) supports vegetarian diets, citing scientific data that suggests an association between a vegetarian diet and a reduced risk for several chronic degenerative diseases and conditions, including obesity, coronary artery disease, hypertension, diabetes, and some types of cancer. It is the position of the ADA that appropriately planned vegetarian diets are healthful, and nutritionally adequate, and provide health benefits in the prevention and treatment of certain diseases.

Some wonder if there is sufficient nutrition in a vegetarian diet to remain fully healthy. But there are many mammals, including cows, elephants, and apes who are by nature 100% raw vegan. These are some of the strongest animals on the planet; they grow strong bones,

**"Desire is the key to motivation, but it's determination and commitment to an unrelenting pursuit of your goal - a commitment to excellence - that will enable you to attain the success you seek."**
~ Mario Andretti

muscle, and develop all the other physiologic components that are needed to be healthy. Also, from what I've learned, the human digestive system is designed best to chemically process food when eating 100% raw vegan food. Doesn't it make sense that this is the best way to eat for long-term good health for all of us?

In *The China Study*, by T. Colin Campbell, Ph.D. and Thomas M. Campbell II, which covers T. Colin Campbell's 25+ year study of nutrition and health, and citing numerous other studies from around the world, the authors state, "Even if you have a high genetic risk, a healthy, plant based diet is capable of negating most, if not all, of that risk by controlling the expression of these genes." (pg. 176). They also state, "Regardless of our genes, we can all optimize our chances of expressing the right genes by providing our bodies with the best possible environment – that is the best possible nutrition." (pg. 235). Knowing information like this can support your commitment to stay on course, even when others ridicule, or harass you, or are uncomfortable with your different eating choices. In addition to self-education, and understanding optimal ways to nourish the human body, how else can we support our commitment?

Creating the best environment for our bodies is supported by creating the best possible environment for our success. We'll delve into some of this a little later, such as associating with others who have chosen this lifestyle, and how to support yourself during the transition phase. Also, it's important to create an environment where you will keep maintaining your actions. I have found several significant tools to help with my journey. To assist in de-stressing, I get regular massage. Also for de-stressing, for over six years now, I've worked with Stillness Technologies, a group that uses a system of breath work, visualization, CDs with vibrational tones, and bodywork to release the long-term effect of stress. This helps create openings for possibility, and allows for more curiosity. Recently, I've read Kurek Ashley's *How Would Love Respond?*, which supports each person's self-empowerment efforts. Finding and using these types of tools will be invaluable in supporting your own journey forward.

## Applying this in your life:

- **Stay curious about what else you can learn about this lifestyle**
- **Explore self-development via books, CDs, events**

Note 1: This is a favorite beverage of mine, my friends and students which I was inspired to create by my visits to Café Gratitude in San Francisco (at the time of this printing, the Café has six locations – each with its own spirit, though all are great to visit!)

Note 2: The added benefit of this drink is that the lemon and the ginger are great digestive enhancements with any meal (best to drink 30 minutes before eating or 1+ hours after eating, to allow your digestive juices to operate maximally)

# NATURAL LEMON GINGERALE

Makes two servings.

Ingredients:
3 lemons
Fresh ginger, about 2 inches
Raw agave nectar
Natural Spring Water (choose the one you like best)

Instructions:
1. Juice the lemons and the fresh ginger together.
2. Pour into two glasses, divided evenly.
3. Add about 2-4 Tablespoons of the agave nectar to each glass, or sweeten to taste (adjusting to your taste after you add the Spring Water).
4. Fill the rest of each glass with the Natural Spring Water, and stir.

The lemon ginger juice will keep in the refrigerator for 3 -4 days.

# Secret #2:

## Allow Time for the Transition

- Recognize Where You Have Gaps
- Be Patient and
- Be Persistent

"Through allowing, you become what you are; vast, spacious. You become whole. You are not a fragment anymore, which is how the ego perceives itself. Your true nature emerges, which is one with the nature of God." ~ Eckhart Tolle

**"The most essential factor is persistence - the determination never to allow your energy or enthusiasm to be dampened by the discouragement that must inevitably come."** ~ James Whitcomb Riley

Have patience with yourself, and persistently continue upon the path you have chosen. So, many of us give up just before achieving success. You are likely to think of at least one instance where you have succeeded when others told you that your goal was impossible, or you have succeeded by applying a more determined focus.

An experience that I had years ago that helped me know that I could make the change to the raw food lifestyle was in my attempts to stop smoking. Yes, I used to smoke cigarettes. As healthy as I am today, many wouldn't ever guess it. I started smoking at age nine, and smoked until I was twenty-three. I quit by sheer will power, though cigarettes still smelled good to me when I'd walk past someone smoking. After three years, I started smoking again. I smoked for another 1 ½ years before I stopped for good. Food can be just as addictive, or more so, as nicotine. Much of the desire for an addictive substance can be tied into our emotions.

From my experience, I have learned that when I continue my focus, even if I have a set-back because of an emotional attachment or desire, I can make a change. I have done it before, and I can do it

**"Nature, time, and patience are the three great physicians."** ~ Proverb quote

again. Knowing this to be true for me, I was able to make it through my stumbles when transitioning to the raw food lifestyle. And, it is a lifestyle. Forget the diets! As the statistics show, for the majority of people, dieting just brings on confusion and a yo-yo, weight loss and gain. Determination, focus of efforts even when stumbling, and some patience will bring you through eventually to your goal.

Give yourself space to make a change. You can even make a game out of small incremental steps to reach your goal. And, when you stumble, acknowledge it, then check in with yourself to see what it was that created a situation where you were willing to step away from your goal, rather than toward your goal. Genuinely recognizing where your slips could occur again is often the biggest step in overcoming the temptation(s).

Food cravings, particularly as your body is getting rid of old, toxic waste from your gut, can sometimes be one of those distractions/temptations. It is frequently a body chemistry reaction, and just needs a minor adjustment on your part to support your goal. See Appendix E at the back of this book for recommendations for some common craving substitutes. These may be helpful in giving you an alternative the next time a craving arises.

You *can* be successful making this change.

"Patience and perseverance have a magical effect before which difficulties disappear and obstacles vanish."
~ John Quincy Adams

Oh, one other thing: If you're like I've been in the past, you might judge yourself for failing in some step. I've learned to forgiveness and love myself, and stick with my focus. A little bit of self-love can go a long way in helping shift your actions!

## Applying this in your life:

1. Breathe
2. Find a quiet spot
3. Find your balance, your center
4. Focus on your goal
5. Set your intention
6. For just a few moments, Do steps 1-5 Daily; even better, do them several times each day.

End of day:
check in with yourself to see where you succeeded, and honestly, where you need more focus/ support/ resources to help you succeed further.

Note: I developed this recipe while healing from oral surgery last Fall, when I was limited to eating soft foods for several weeks. It has become a favorite, especially since it's so easy to put together.

# CORN CHOWDER

Makes two servings.

Ingredients:
2 C Corn kernels, preferably fresh (can use organic frozen or dehydrated as well; with dehydrated, soak in your soup water)
2 C purified water (can be the soak water for the dehydrated corn)
3 stalks celery
1 avocado
1 tsp sea salt
1 tsp onion powder
1 tsp cumin
Paprika, for appearance
Fresh Ground Black Pepper, to taste

Instructions:
1. Reserve ¼ C of the corn kernels on the side. Blend all remaining ingredients together in a blender until smooth. Can blend it to warmth, though be careful of blending it too hot, or will kill the enzymes.
2. By hand, stir in the remaining corn kernels.
3. Pour into serving bowls.
4. Sprinkle top with paprika and a touch of fresh ground black pepper.

This will keep the refrigerator for about two days.

# Secret #3:

## <u>Variety IS the Spice of Life</u>

- Own Your Options

"I am a possibilist. I believe that humanity is master of its own fate... Before we can change direction, we have to question many of the assumptions underlying our current philosophy. Assumptions like bigger is better; …. Then we have to replace them with some different assumptions: small is beautiful; roots and traditions are worth preserving; variety is the spice of life; the only work worth doing is meaningful work; biodiversity is the necessary pre-condition for human survival." ~ Robert Bateman

**"You have to eat a variety of different foods to get all the nutrients your body needs to keep you healthy. By eating the same thing day after day you won't get these protective nutrients."**
~ Dee Murphy

With variety in your choices, you have fun and enjoy this food journey, this exploration in what can be one of the most rewarding ways to live.

I am grateful my parents had eclectic and adventuresome tastes when it came to food. They only required that my older brother and I at least taste the food before we could say definitively that we didn't like it. I've heard stories where parents would force their kids to "eat all your veggies, 'cause it's good for you,"; though they'd serve veggies so overcooked, who could find them palatable? Consequently, some of these children have sometimes grown up thinking that they don't like vegetables.

Recently in one of my classes, a student who determined to make the transition to raw foods for her long-term health. She thought she didn't like veggies, and was thinking about going to a hypnotist for help on this. I encouraged her to wait, and experience the lifestyle for a while before spending the money. After tasting the recipes from the class, she stated that she was surprised that she liked everything except one item, and that it seemed as if the freshness and the spices made all the difference. She departed the class excited by experiencing a whole new world of

**"Our minds are like our stomachs; they are whetted by the change of their food, and variety supplies both with fresh appetites."**
~ John Quinton

possibilities opening before her, and relief from realizing that this was going to be easier than she had thought.

If you truly find that you don't like vegetables, you can effectively eat raw as a fruitarian; though balance and high sugar are challenges. Most important, however you choose to implement the raw food lifestyle, make sure to change up your meals. This variety serves two purposes.

The first purpose is to keep the lifestyle evolving and interesting for you, so that you stay committed to eating the best way you can. The second purpose is for your health. When continually eating the same foods over and over, you can build up food allergies, intolerances, as well as experience gaps in your nutritional needs. The variety mix is recommended to ensure that you are getting balanced nutrition naturally.

Raw food lifestyle choices include fruitarian, Ayurvedic/Phase style as taught by Gabriel Cousens, MD; high raw as taught by Fred Bisci and Frederick Patenaude; gourmet/high raw as taught by Cherie Soria; 80/10/10 as taught by Doug Graham, DC, which is geared toward athletes as advocated by Graham and also Brendan Brazier. And, if you're looking for help with healing a health crisis, either Cousens' Tree of Life in Patagonia, Arizona, the Hippocrates Institute in West

**"Variety's the very spice of life, That gives it all its flavor"** ~ William Cowper

Palm Beach, Florida or the Gerson Institute now in Mexico, can be helpful; all three incorporate juice fasting as part of their healing assistance. An on-site coach to walk you through initial changes can be of invaluable assistance, especially if this is a critical life change that you're looking to implement.

You can see that there are quite a few ways to implement the raw or high raw lifestyle. Connect with the one that's right for you and your body. You learn what is right for your body by experimenting, exploring the variety of options in the beginning. See which one, or combination, you resonate with the most. Ask yourself, as you experiment, "How does this impact allergies that I've had, my weight, my sleep? Does it help me to feel energetic and vibrant? " These are good questions to continue to ask yourself as you go forward, since the body's needs are always changing.

## Applying this in your life:

- **Start by exploring the variety of ways to adopt the raw food lifestyle.**
- **Make sure that you are getting a variety of items in your meals each week, for both your interest and your good health.**

Note 1: This is a modification of a recipe from Gabriel Cousens' *Rainbow Green Live-Food Cuisine*, p. 250

Note 2: For a meal, this is especially nice in contrast with a living foods Chili (I particularly like the *Unbelievable Chili* recipe from Angela Elliott's *Alive in 5* ); it has become a favorite winter meal.

Note 3: I enjoy pairing this salad with Enchiladas or Burritos or Tacos, for a Mexican inspired meal. It's great any time of year, since it's light and refreshing.

Note 4: This will keep in the refrigerator for 2-3 days, though for optimal nutrition, it is best eaten freshly made.

# ZEN CABBAGE SALAD

Ingredients:
2 C green cabbage
¼ C sesame seeds
1 ½ T sesame oil
2 tsp lemon juice
¼ tsp ginger juice [optional]
¾ tsp sea salt

Instructions:
1. Combine cabbage and salt in a good size mixing bowl.
2. Massage the salt into the cabbage.
3. Let it sit for 10 minutes.
4. Add remaining ingredients and mix well.

# Secret #4:

## Spices Keep it Fun

"Spice is life. It depends upon what you like... have fun with it. Yes, food is serious, but you should have fun with it. ~ Emeril Lagasse

**"There is no single face in nature, because every eye that looks upon it, sees it from its own angle. So every man's spice-box seasons his own food."**
~ Zora Neale Hurston

I can only speak for myself, and speaking for myself, I demand two criteria of my food. First, I desire vibrant food that looks gorgeous on the plate, proving irresistible and tempting the palate. Second, I expect food to smell great and taste wonderful. Why settle for less, when you can get all of this? And, the fact that it's so nutritious and healthy just makes it all that much more attractive!

Spice can be one of the most fun parts of experiencing raw foods. It helps elevate food from the mundane to the sublime. In the culinary arts, flavorings are a good part of what makes up 'gastronomy'. According to Merriam-Webster's on-line dictionary, gastronomy is the art or science of good eating.

Spices keep it fun and interesting. Here is an opportunity to experiment and find new things that you like. One fun thing you can do is play with food like we did at the Living Light Culinary Arts Institute. For one of our sessions, we were provided with toothpicks, and small cups of various items that fit into the six flavor groups: Sweet, Salty, Tart, Pungent, Bitter, and Fat. We then created mixtures of these (for flavor balancing, you'll want to include at least one item from each group) to see what we liked. For example, one

that I put together and liked was Agave,
Dark miso, Pineapple, Onion powder,
Kale, and Tahini; another was Apple,
Celery, Tamarind, Green Onion and
Mustard (both pungents), Basil, and
Coconut Oil.

And, remember, your flavoring
preferences might be different from
someone else's.  Also, please be aware that
the young and the old are more sensitive
to spice than many others.  When you
have guests, keep this in mind when you
prepare your foods.

Spices and herbs have played a key role in
the historical development of civilization.
Spices today are widely available and are
used mostly as flavorings. However, up
until the 1900s, they were highly prized
products, used for medicine, perfume,
incense, and flavoring.  Our love affair
with spices continues. Today we have the
spices of the world at our fingertips and
we use them to create the dishes of many
cultures. We also continue to be interested
in their medicinal value.  I'll touch on the
medicinal aspects a little more in the next
section when we talk about detoxification.

The great and wonderful thing about
spices for the raw food lifestyle is that you
can take the same base recipe and create a
very different taste experience with it, just
by changing the spices.  A good example
is a nut or seed pate that can be flavored

**" When we share meals ...We try to ensure
that our main courses present a variety of
textures, colors, and flavors, balance our
affinity for sweet and sour and satisfy our
taste for salt and spice."** ~ Matthew
Kenney and Sarma Melngailis from *Raw
Food, real world*

to taste like an Italian dish, or a Japanese
dish, or a dish from India, depending on
the spices you use. Chef Chad Sarno, put
together a great resource for working with
spices and creating different ethnic based
flavor combinations (see his booklet
information in Appendix B in the back of
this book). Using his chart, it is easy to
put together all sorts of dishes, letting
your imagination and taste buds play with
the flavors you like to create something
totally new, or to adjust a recipe that
you've made and feel needs something
more for your palate.

Most importantly, check out the variety of
spices available, and see what fun you can
have creating new and interesting
combinations. If you are like me,
admittedly, some dishes you make will fall
short of meeting your expectations. On
the other hand, you'll come up with some
outstanding dishes that you can proudly
share with others. The spices can
invigorate your life by adding variety and
new ideas.

## Applying this in your life:
- **Experiment with flavors**
- **Play with your food!**

Note 1: This recipe was created by Amanda Crook, my instructor for Alissa Cohen's Raw Chef certification. She said her inspiration came from Alissa Cohen's Sour Cream recipe.

Note 2: At home, I make Igor Boutenko's Live Flat Bread, and use this onion dip as a sandwich spread, with sliced avocadoes, sundried tomatoes, and lettuce, and sometimes sprouts.

Note 3: This makes a great party dip, with celery, and carrot sticks, and zucchini rounds.

Note 4: This dip will last about a week in the refrigerator.

# AMANDA'S ONION DIP

Ingredients:
1 ½ C cashews
3 T apple cider vinegar
1 ½ tsp mellow white miso
1 t sea salt
1/8 tsp cayenne (optional)
Juice of a lemon
½ C water, or less
1 clove garlic, pressed
1 C onions, minced
¼ - ½ C chives, minced (optional)
[recommended]

Instructions:
1. In a Vita-Mix blender or other blender or food processor, blend the cashews, vinegar, miso, salt, cayenne and lemon juice. Slowly add water until smooth and creamy. (Start with ½ C water and add more only if needed to make the mixture blend. Keep this as thick as you can, and make sure it's as smooth and creamy as possible when done.)
2. Remove mixture from the blender/processor, and add in by hand the garlic, onions and chives. Mix gently and chill.

# Secret #5:

## <u>Detoxification Experiences Can Help Your Transition</u>

- Adjust your intake to your comfort level

**"Excess generally causes reaction, and produces a change in the opposite direction, whether it be in the seasons, or in individuals, or in governments."**
~ Plato

**"Spiritual progress is like detoxification. Things have to come up in order to be released. Once we have asked to be healed, then our unhealed places are forced to the surface."**
~ Marianne Williamson

It is truly wonderful if you avoid experiencing the symptoms of detoxification; some people go slowly enough that all they feel is the energy gain from the lifestyle change. Many of us changing over, myself included, have experienced some initial short-term discomforts from the detoxification. Personally, I celebrated the release. It was worth a little discomfort to know that I was healing my body. I invite you to shift your perception similarly.

Most of us have spent a life-time putting foods and chemicals into our bodies that disagree with the balance of the natural human system. When a person begins the process of cleaning up their food intake, they can reasonably expect some degree of detoxification reaction. I did, even though I was a vegetarian for almost ten years prior to making this life change, and I had done all kinds of liver and kidney cleanses, and colonics, and herbs. Others that I know and have worked with have too – it's fairly typical. The degree of detoxification depends upon you.

Some people start to get gas and/or indigestion, and think that this way of eating isn't working for them. What is actually happening is that the body is finally getting some relief from all of the chemicals and toxins previously being put

**"Our body's natural detoxification system is designed to support our health by eliminating waste products from our metabolism and from environmental toxins."** ~ Mark Hyman

into the body, and is beginning to release some of the build up in the tissues.

Other symptoms of detoxification can include stomach grumbling, tiredness, and headaches. If you continue to eat well, and drink enough pure water to help flush the toxins, these symptoms should pass within a few days, or a week at the most.

Be aware that you have control over the speed and intensity of your reaction. Fast detoxification can cause severe reactions, such as migraine headaches, nausea, constipation, or diarrhea. Also, if you are dealing with a severe illness such as cancer or diabetes, I highly recommend that you only take on detoxification while working with a knowledgeable health practitioner, like Dr. Gabriel Cousens' group at the Tree of Life Rejuvenation Center in Arizona, the Hippocrates Health Institute in Florida, or the Gerson Institute in Mexico.

You can slow down this process by eating the denser food choices available, especially those containing fats, such as avocados and nuts and seeds. Additionally, know that "food combining" can play an important role here. It's best to keep it simple. Since lighter foods and beverages, such as smoothies or melons or simple meals of salad greens or fruit, digest faster than denser, heavier foods,

**"Action and reaction, ebb and flow, trial and error, change - this is the rhythm of living. Out of our over-confidence, fear; out of our fear, clearer vision, fresh hope. And out of hope, progress."**
~ Bruce Barton

such as nuts and seeds and avocados, always eat the lighter items first or even solo. Otherwise, the lighter, faster digesting item(s) sit(s) on top of the heavier, slower digesting item(s), creating fermentation and thereby giving you gas and intestinal discomfort, in addition to being a stress on your body's systems.

Several herbs can also be of assistance in soothing the tummy, or alleviating headaches, or tiredness. For gas, add dill, fennel, peppermint, catsnip, or sweet marjoram. For tiredness, rosemary, basil, and several essential oils in aromatherapy can help. I carry a high-quality line of essential oils, and can guide you in exploring how essential oils can help. For indigestions, chamomile, ginger, and peppermint are well known resources. And, for headaches, lavender and peppermint oil aromatherapy, and feverfew or willow can be very helpful.

## Applying this in your life:
- **Plan a low-stress week the 1st week you make your transition**
- **Support your body with rest, herbs, and aromatherapy**

Note 1:  This sauce is my modified
version of Alissa Cohen's *Living On
Live Food*,  Marinara Sauce, pg. 367.

Note 2 : in place of the 12 sundried
tomatoes and ¼ C olive oil, I often
use 1 jar of Mediterranean Organic
sundried tomatoes in olive oil.  For
those on the go, this can be a time
saver.

# PASTA MARINARA

Ingredients:
2 zucchini, med. Size
1 pint box of cherry tomatoes
12 sundried tomatoes, soaked
¼ C olive oil
4 cloves garlic
5-7 black mission figs (can be dried, though soak to plump prior to use)
2 T parsley
2-3 T basil (adjusted to your tastes)
1/16 tsp cayenne
¾ tsp sea salt
Gopal's Rawmesan Cheese (optional)
Pine Nuts (optional)

Instructions:
1. Place all ingredients, except the zucchini, in a food processor, and blend to the consistency you like for spaghetti sauce.
2. Rinse the zucchini, and cut off both tips. Then make noodles from these, in one of two ways: a) use a Spirooli or Spiralizer to make thin angel hair type pasta, or b) use a vegetable peeler to make long strips lengthwise from the zucchini.
3. Place the noodles on plates, and pour the sauce over top. Then, sprinkle the top with Gopal's Rawmesan Cheese and Pine Nuts; can also add chopped olives, or other ingredients you like in your spaghetti.

# Secret #6:

## <u>Seek Continued Support</u>

- Learn new techniques and options to keep you interested
- Fine-tune your skills and knowledge

**"They understand they don't have all the answers. It's good to always seek knowledge and they always ask good questions. They always ask, 'What am I not doing?' or 'What do you see that I'm not seeing?' "** ~ Howard Moore

**"The only people who achieve much are those who want knowledge so badly that they seek it while the conditions are still unfavourable. Favourable conditions never come."**
~ C.S. Lewis

Continue to seek additional support and resources, whether it is through books, websites, links, forums, raw food potlucks, or other groups that will support your choices.

Being focused on, and surrounding yourself with whatever you wish to create in your life is a KEY ACTION in supporting your choices. Success is yours with the action taken.

As a starter, refer to the Appendices A through D which include books, links and resources that can offer particular help in transitioning to the raw food lifestyle.

Recall again Secret #1: Your commitment to this lifestyle and associating with others who have chosen this lifestyle can be an invaluable support. This is important enough to repeat again. We become like the influences around us; as the influences contain our focus, our focus creates our thought patterns, and in turn, our thought patterns create our actions and environment.

Association with others who have chosen this lifestyle can be especially helpful when you are in the transition phase. Once the lifestyle is in place, then the associations can continue just for the

**"The greatest influence in your life, stronger even than your will power, is your environment. Change that, if necessary."** ~ Paramahansa Yogananda

pleasure of it, if you so choose.

How can you associate with others, especially if you are far from a big city? On-line, there are several groups, on Facebook, and Yahoo! Groups, or and some of the teachers are also accessible. For example, Alissa Cohen has a raw food forum via her website (see resource guide in the back of this book for the address). This can be fun and educational, as people come from all levels of experience and share new recipes, and ideas. If you are in a larger town or city, many have pot-luck or meet-up groups for people at least interested in exploring this lifestyle. Staying curious and open, and checking out how and what others are doing as an expression of their raw food lifestyle, can give you new ideas, help keep your focus, and continually refresh your commitment.

From personal experience, I know that reaching out, and asking for help, can be difficult sometimes. One strategy I find helpful is to use index cards with affirmation statements on them. These contain the thoughts and actions that I wish to keep at the forefront of my focus. I've done this off and on since the late 1980s. When I do use them, life just seems to be better, more focused, and going in the direction that I truly choose. I repeat these affirmations each morning to help set the tone of my day. This is a

**"The truth is that is doesn't matter what you want in your life – the strategies are the same. You have to open up your mind to accept some concepts that may be new to you because it's the only way your life is going to transform to the next level."**
~ Kurek Ashley

way that you can receive help from your best self. And, if you find it difficult to receive help from others, you can write an affirmation to support your receiving help easily. Always write your affirmation in the present tense to instill it in your subconscious mind. This will ensure that your affirmation comes to exist in the world.

## Applying this in your life:

- **Reach out for the success you seek by surrounding yourself with others who are successful doing what you wish to do.**
- **Support your commitment via association with others that have chosen this lifestyle:**
  - **Join an on-line group**
  - **Join or create a local pot-luck or meet-up group**
- **Use affirmations**

Note 1 : These recipes come directly from Brigitte Mars' *Rawsome!*, pg. 179 and pg. 184; this book also contains a great Raw Food Encyclopedia in the front section.

Note 2 : I love serving these as a side dish with Brigitte's Kale Salad recipe, and Gabriel Cousens' Dahl recipe from *Rainbow Green Live-Food Cuisine*.

## MASHED PARSNIPS

By Brigitte Mars; Yield: 4-6 servings

Ingredients:
1 C macadamia nuts, soaked overnight,
then rinsed
8 parsnips, peeled and chopped (about 6 C)
1 C water
1 tsp sea salt
¼ tsp fresh ground black pepper

Instructions: Combine all ingredients in a
food processor (or blender for a smoother
consistency), and blend until the mixture
is thick and smooth.

⇨Serve this dish with Nama Shoyu Gravy

▤Can substitute rutabaga for the parsnips, if
desired.


with


## NAMA SHOYU GRAVY

Yield: 1 C

Ingredients:
¼ C olive oil
¼ C Nama Shoyu
¼ C nutritional yeast (optional; not a raw
product)
¼ C water

Instructions: Combine all ingredients in a
blender and blend until smooth.

# Secret #7:

## <u>Follow Your Own Body's Guidance</u>

- Take your action steps from here.

**"We don't need someone to show us the ropes. We are the ones we've been waiting for. Deep inside us we know the feelings we need to guide us. Our task is to learn to trust our inner knowing."** ~ Sonia Johnson

**"What lies behind us and what lies before us are small matters compared to what lies within us."** ~ Ralph Waldo Emerson

You are your own greatest Guide in what works best for you. I remind each individual I work with that each person has unique needs, coming from different backgrounds, and different health points. To learn what is working best for you, it is very important for you to listen for the clues from your own body. Also, remember that this will change over time. For example, when I first began eating raw foods, I felt that I needed the heavier, denser foods in order to feel full. After six months of eating 100% raw (part of which was doing a 60-day juice fast to clean out my body). I started getting digestive upsets every few days. I noticed that this occurred after I ate the meals with the heavier, denser foods. When I started eliminating these heavier items from my regular meals, I felt better and slept better once again.

This isn't to say that I never eat a meal containing these items now; I just limit them to special occasions and some winter meals. My body tells me, by how I feel in my gut, and how I process and eliminate foods, how well the foods that I eat are working for me.

I do have a caveat to this advice: when you first change over to raw foods, you may find it a challenge to understand what your body is telling you, since you've

"Your time is limited, so don't waste it living someone else's life. Don't be trapped by dogma - which is living with the results of other people's thinking. Don't let the noise of others' opinions drown out your own inner voice. And most important, have the courage to follow your heart and intuition. They somehow already know what you truly want to become. Everything else is secondary."
~ Steve Jobs

possibly been eating (meat and cooked foods) out of alignment with your natural body chemistry. With commitment and patience, and allowing time to get through the initial adjustments, you soon get a sense of what is working and not working for your body. I recommend giving the initial change over at least 30 days before evaluating the effect of what is happening within your body, on your attitudes, and in your life.

If you are eating well-balanced, raw vegan meals, it is highly likely that you will begin to eat less over time. Your body will be able to benefit from the wealth of nutrition that raw food offers, and you just don't need as much. Your transition meals are likely to be quite different from the meals that you will be drawn to in six months, a year, or many years later.

It is also likely that your metabolism and digestion will start to align with the natural rhythms of the planet, with the circadian rhythms that govern the ebb and flow of the daily rhythmic activity cycle. As you change your eating, you'll probably notice that your digestion is best during mid-day.

**"You are always your own best guru, your own best teacher, the answers are always inside you."** ~ Sai Baba

In the Ayurvedic system from India, a health system around for several thousands of years, the 24-hour day is split into cycles supporting the strength of different parts of the body, and digestion is considered the strongest between 10 a.m. and 2 p.m. With this consideration, to support your best digestion and body assimilation, your heaviest meal of the day, and perhaps eventually your only meal of the day, would be during that time frame.

As you go forward, you will live life based more on your own internal experience. Flavors will be different at different times. Trust what you are attracted to. Honor it. Act on it.

Finally, doing it all with love in your heart will make the food taste better for you, and for those with whom you choose to share your food journey. Enjoy!

## Applying this in your life:
- **Start by listening within to understand what is best for you.**
- **ACT: Change only happens when you take action, so ACT on what you know!**

Note: These are wonderful little treats for those with a sweet tooth, especially those who adore chocolate; I found this recipe in *The Complete Book of Raw Food*, a great compendium from many living food chefs.

# HAYSTACKS

By Elaina Love; Yields: 20 pcs

Ingredients:
¾ C coconut oil
½ C agave nectar or honey or other natural raw sweetener
½ C organic cacao powder or carob powder
1 tsp vanilla extract or 1/8 vanilla bean
3 C shredded coconut (more or less as needed)

Instructions:
1. In a blender add liquefied coconut oil, agave nectar, cacao or carob powder, and vanilla. If using a vanilla bean, cut the bean open and use the black pulp inside. Blend on high until the batter emulsifies.
2. Mix the batter with the shredded coconut n a large mixing bowl.
3. Form the haystack shapes on a tray lined with wax paper. Let these set in the refrigerator or freezer before serving. The haystacks will be soft at temperatures over 60 degrees F; they'll last 6-12 months in the refrigerator or freezer (if you don't eat them first)

# APPENDIX A
## Some Favorite Raw Recipe Books include (alpha listing by author's last name):

* **Living in the Raw** by Rose Lee Calabro (particularly good bread and cracker recipes)

* **Conscious Eating** by Gabriel Cousens, MD (recipes categorized by Ayurvedic body type)

* **Rainbow Green Live-Food Cuisine** by Gabriel Cousens, MD (in-depth medical-scientific basis and data, plus balanced for health recipes, with plans for clearing and eating according to Ayurvedic body type)

* **Alive in 5** by Angela Elliott

* **I Am Grateful** by Terces Engelhart with Orchid (by the creator of Café Gratitude in San Francisco)

* **everyday raw** by Matthew Kenney (NYC Chef extraordinaire; see his website link in next section to see what he's creating now)

* **RAW FOOD real world** by Matthew Kenney and Sarma Melngailis

* **Elaina's Pure Joy Kitchen #2** by Elaina Love

* **RAWSOME!** by Brigitte Mars (a great resource for both tasty recipes, as well as a helpful raw food encyclopedia in the front of the book)

* **Raw Spirit** by Matt Monarch

* **How We All Went Raw** by Charles, Coralanne, and George Nungesser (a well done spiral bound booklet, with quite a few different and tasty recipes)

* **ani's raw food kitchen** by Ani Phyo

* **Vital Creations** by Chad Sarno (a great resource for those looking to create some of their own dishes; includes a chart of common spices by ethnic food groups, plus other helpful suggestions)

* **The Raw Food Revolution Diet** by Cherie Soria, Brenda Davis, ,RD, and Vesanto Melina, MS, RD

* **Living Cuisine** by Renee Loux Underkoffler

# APPENDIX B
## Additional Related Book Resources include (alpha listing by author's last name):

* **Cleanse & Purify Thyself** by Richard Anderson, ND., NMD

* **Alkalize or Die** by Theodore A. Baroody, ND, DC, PhD nutrition, CNC

* **The China Study** by T. Collin Campbell, PhD, and Thomas M. Campbell, II

* **Mucusless Diet Healing System** and **Rational Fasting** by Professor Arnold Ehret

* **Diet for a New America** by John Robbins

* **The Live Food Factor** by Susan Schenck, LAc, MTOM

* **Become Younger** and **Fresh Vegetable and Fruit Juices** by Dr. N.W. Walker, DSc

# APPENDIX C
## Some Interesting and Helpful Raw Resource Websites include (alpha listing by first letter of website domain name) :

* http://tinyurl.com/kwu75t (link to the **Vibrant Living Expo and Culinary Showcase**, a production, organized by Living Light International and the Institute for Vibrant Living)

* www. alissacohen.com (raw food forum, store with resources, and more)

* http://apps.ams.usda.gov/FarmersMarkets/ (to find local Farmers Markets)

* www. aulac.com (Menu and location for Chef Ito)

* www. brendanbrazier.com (Brendan Brazier's site; great resource for athletes)

* www. E3live.com (complete nutrition green food supplements to help you energize, focus, and balance – considered one of the best on the market)

* www.excaliburdehydrator.com (often considered the best food

dehydrator, and raw food industry standard)

* www.ezjuicers.com (the single auger style units will help retain more of the food enzymes)

* www. fredbisci4health.com (Fred Bisci's site; advocate of the Healthy Journey Experience, conferences and products)

* www. fredericpatenaude.com (enewsletter, blog, articles, programs, and more)

* www.gerson.org (dedicated to the holistic treatment of degenerative diseases)

* www.glaserorganicfarms.com (can get some raw food items here)

* www.gliving.tv/greenchefs/ (internet TV site offering some chefs sharing raw food ideas)

* www.hippocratesinst.com (Hippocrates Health Institute – West Palm Beach, Florida)

* www.thelaughinggiraffe.com (a few select yummy treats and granolas)

* www.living-foods.com (a well established raw food networking and resource site)

* www.livingtreecommunity.com (a community providing quite a few nuts, seeds, butters, oils, and supplies; often purchase supplies here)

* www. matthewkenney.com (Matthew Kenney's news site)

* http: tinyurl.com/nhgxx3 (Site offering well-priced raw foods and supportive supplies for a raw food lifestyle – one I return to again and again)

* www.oneluckyduck.com (Sarma Melngailis' resource site)

* www.paulnison.com (Paul Nison's site; raw food author and lecturer)

* www.purejoylivingfoods.com (Elaina Love's site; raw food author and lecturer, chef, and instructor)

* www.rawbakery.com

* www. rawchef.org (Chad Sarno's site; classes, books, chef training in England)

* www. rawfamily.com (the Boutenko family's site; enewsletter, books, and more)

* www.rawfood.com (Nature's First Law Raw Food site)

* www.rawfoodchef.com (Living Light Culinary Arts Institute site)

* www.rawfoodinfo.com (Rhio's site; see her list of raw restaurants, take out, and juice bars)

* www.rawfoodsnewsmagazine.com

* www.rawfoodtalk.com/forum (Alissa Cohen's site and raw food forum)

* www.rawfromthefarm.com (a farm and group providing well-priced fresh supplies, nuts, seeds, green powders, and items; another one that I often return to for supplies)

* www.rawganique.com (offering a variety of raw resources)

* www. rawgourmet.com (Nomi Shannon's site; enewsletter, and more)

* www. rawmmgood.com (my site; classes, chef training, enewsletter, and resources)

\* www. rawspirit.org (Matt Monarch's site; The Raw Food World enewsletter, store with resources, and more)

\* www.rawveganbooks.com (a resource for a multiple of items, in addition to books, related to supporting a raw food lifestyle – site with great offerings)

\* www. renegadehealth.com (Kevin Gianni's site, with an enewsletter, and all sorts of good information and resources)

\* www.sunorganicfarms.com (some raw food items available here)

\* www.treeoflife.nu (Site for Gabriel Cousens' community and offerings)

\* www.ulimana.com (awesome chocolate treats for those who will still eat chocolate)

\* www.vitamix.com (sells highly durable and versatile blender; a raw food industry standard)

\* www. welikeitraw.com (keeps up with raw lifestyle related videos)

# APPENDIX D
## Other Interesting and Helpful Resource Websites to Support a Raw Lifestyle:

(alpha listing by first letter of website domain name)

* http://tinyurl.com/n7mbuu
**(Everything Is Energy, Prosperity Tribe** – a powerful program, hosted and led by the Morellis; assists in releasing blocks to achieve financial independence)

* www.coopamerica.com (E-newsletter – Green America, and more)

* www.Envirosax.com (really cool, well designed reusable bags)

* www.howwouldloverespond.com (Kurek Ashley's site for his book, *How Would Love Respond?*, events, and additional resources; great resources for personal empowerment)

* www.idealbite.com (Earth friendly ideas shared via daily email tidbit)

* www.lifekind.com (organic and natural bedding, and cleaning products)

* www.LivinginStillness.com (Stillness Technologies; helped me greatly in opening to new possibilities, and learning how to stay curious about life)

* www.Peacefulcompany.com
(Eco friendly products and gifts)

* www.roadfood.com   (to find
organic food across the country)

* www.to-goware.com   (innovative
utensils, containers, and products that
provide a solution, tell a great story, and
are enjoyable to use)

* www.tspspices.com   (organic spices
in teaspoon size packets; great for travel —
a thoughtful gift to me originally by Kathy
Kamisky of Davis, California)

# APPENDIX E
# If you have cravings, for some not-so-healthy foods, here are healthy alternates:

♦**Acid foods or Chocolate**
Your body calling may be for added:
•**Magnesium** - apricots, avocados, bananas, broccoli, cantaloupe, carrots, cauliflower, celery, dandelion greens, dates, figs, dark leafy greens (esp. beet, collard, mustard, spinach, Swiss Chard), mangoes, nuts (esp. almonds, Brazil, cashew, pecan , pine nuts, walnuts), oranges, paprika, parsley, parsnips, peaches, peppermint

♦**Alcohol, recreational drugs**
•**Protein** – algaes (esp. super blue-greens like E3live, or Spirulina), dark leafy greens, hemp seeds, nuts
•**Calcium** – almonds, Brazil nuts, broccoli, carob, dandelion greens, dark leafy greens (esp. collard, mustard, turnip, kale), figs, miso, hazelnuts, seaweeds (esp. dulse, kelp, hiziki, kombu, wakame), sesame seeds, sunflower seeds
•**Glutamine** – cabbage juice, parsley, spinach
•**Potassium** – almonds, apricots, avocados, bananas, beets, blueberries, buckwheat, cabbages, cantaloupe, carrots, dandelion greens, dates, dulse, figs, garlic, grapes/raisins, dark leafy greens (esp. beet, spinach, Swiss Chard), onions, oranges, papayas, peaches, pumpkin seeds, sage, seaweeds, sundried black olives, sunflower seeds, tomatoes, watermelon, winter squash

## ♦Bread
•**Nitrogen** – algae's (esp. super blue-greens like E3live, or Spirulina), dark leafy greens, hemp seeds, nuts

## ♦Coffee or Tea
•**Phosphorous** – broccoli, garlic, dark leafy greens (esp. collard, kale), nuts (esp. almonds), parsnips, pumpkin seeds, sesame seeds, seaweeds (esp. dulse)
/•**Sulfur** – apples, apricots, blue-green algae (such as E3live), broccoli, cabbages, carrots, cauliflower, cayenne, celery, durians, garlic, dark leafy greens (esp. kale, mustard, Swiss Chard), hemp seeds, nuts (all), onions, peaches, plums/prunes, Spirulina, turnips
•**Sodium** – apples, apricots, beets, coconut, celery, dandelion greens, grapes/raisins, olives, seaweeds, sesame seeds, strawberries, sweet potatoes, turnips, Himalayan or Celtic Sea Salt
•**Iron** – almonds, apricots, blackberries, carrots, cherries, dandelion greens, deep-colored fruit, grapes/raisins, dark leafy greens (esp. collard, kale, spinach, Swiss Chard), seaweed

## ♦Fatty foods or snacks
•**Calcium** – see list above in "Alcohol" craving

## ♦General Overeating
• **Silicon** – almonds, apples, apricots, asparagus, beets, carrots, cauliflower, celery cherries, cucumber, dandelion greens, figs grapes/raisins, hemp seeds, horseradish, kelp, leafy greens (esp. lettuce, spinach, Swiss Chard), parsnips, peppers, pumpkins, radishes, sprouts (esp.

alfalfa), strawberries, sunflower seeds, tomatoes, watermelon

•**Tryptophan** – avocados, bananas, chives, dates, durians, figs, grapefruit, nuts (esp. cashews), oranges, papayas, peaches, pears, pineapple, seeds (esp. pumpkin, sunflower), strawberries, tomatoes

•**Tyrosine** – almonds, apples, apricots, avocados, bananas, beets, bell peppers, carrots, cherries, cucumbers, figs, lettuce, parsley, pumpkin seeds, sesame seeds, sunflower seeds, spinach, Spirulina, strawberries, watermelon

◆**PMS** (Premenstrual Syndrome)

•**Zinc** – alfalfa sprouts, almonds, bee pollen, Brazil nuts, cashews, cayenne, chamomile, coconut, dandelion greens, garlic, fennel seeds, kelp leafy green vegetables (esp. spinach), macadamia nuts, nutritional yeast, onions, parsley, pecans, sage, sesame seeds, sunflower seeds, walnuts

◆**Sodas**

•**Calcium** – see list above in "Alcohol craving

◆**Sweets**

•**Chromium** – apples, bananas, basil, beets, broccoli, black pepper, carrots, grapes/raisins, nuts (esp. walnuts)

•**Phosphorus** – see "Coffee or Tea" list

•**Sulfur** – see "Coffee or Tea" list above

•**Tryptophan** – see "General Overeating" list above

◆**Tobacco**

•**Silicon** – see "General Overeating" list

•**Tyrosine** – see " General Overeating"

"Cravings" List Source Information:

1. Benard Jenson, PhD. *The Chemistry of Man* B. Jensen Publisher, 1983
2. Brigitte Mars, *RAWSOME!*, Basic Health Publications, Inc., 2004

# Recipe
# Bibliography

Zen Cabbage:
Cousens, MD, Gabriel, *Rainbow
Green Live-Food Cuisine*, Berkeley,
California, North Atlantic Books
and Patagonia, Arizona, Essene
Vision Books, 2003

Pasta Marinara:
Cohen, Alissa, *Living On Live Food*,
Laguna Beach, California, Cohen
Publishing Company, 2004

Mashed Parsnips and
Nama Shoyu Gravy:
Mars, Brigitte, *RAWSOME!*,
Laguna Beach, California, Basic
Health Publications, Inc., 2004

Haystacks:
Love, Elaina, Pure Joy Kitchen
Recipe Binder #2, Pure Joy Living
Foods
[ www.purejoylivingfoods.com ]

# YOUR NOTES:

Breinigsville, PA USA
28 September 2009
224852BV00001B/9/P